All The Shit They

Don't Tell You

Pregnancy + Motherhood

This book is dedicated to my daughter Ava Love, you are my greatest decision and adventure. Thank you for making me a mommy.

And to all the Mother's and Mother's to be: You can be a mess and still be a good mom.

Table Of Contents

PART 1

INTRODUCTION

I was young when my parents divorced. My father gained custody over my two brothers and I. It wasn't common to see a young man raising three kids on his own in the '90s. Let alone in the big city of Atlanta. In order to support his family, my father worked long hours. This left a lot of responsibility on me because I was the oldest. I became the "woman" of the house at an early age (whether I liked it or not). Because my dad was always working, I would be left "in charge." Unbeknownst to me, I was gaining a good sense of what adulthood would be like early on. Before the age of ten, I was responsible for doing the laundry, making sure my brothers ate, ensuring the house was cleaned, and verifying all homework was done. Around four o'clock every morning my dad would wake me up early (while my brothers were still sleeping) to walk him to the front door. He would make sure I locked up the house properly when it was time for him to leave for work. I would then lay in bed waiting for my alarm clock to go off to make sure we all made it to school on time.

I think this is where my anxiety began. Having too much responsibility at an early age can have lasting effects on a young child. As I got older and began growing into a young woman, I told myself I would not be responsible for anyone else. My dad did the best he could but watching him struggle to take care of his children, made me vow to never have kids of my own. I just wanted to be responsible for me, myself, and I. I had been helping raise kids since I was a kid. So, I made myself my only obligation.

When I turned twenty, I started dating my high school crush. Before you know it, twenty-four months later, I was married. I married a great man who at the time had a young daughter. If I'm truthful, I was hesitant because I was young and had no desire to raise kids. However, I fell in love with the both of them and the rest is now history. Throughout our marriage, I was constantly asked by family and friends "when are you guys going to have kids?" They would say, "It's about time to have some babies." I felt drained constantly saying the same thing over and over "I don't plan on having kids." I always knew my husband wanted more children. He asked me for many years to have at least one child. But I was very clear and frank in expressing my desire not to have any. I could see in his eyes that my decision crushed his spirit. But he eventually adjusted, and life went on. There's a saying that the older and wiser folks like to say: If you want to make God laugh tell him about your plans.

I don't know what happened but seven years into our marriage at age twenty-nine my biological clock felt like it started working overtime. The desire of wanting to create life within me and have that feeling of unconditional love had become overwhelming. Where did this come from? And why NOW?! Lol! My stepdaughter at that time was eleven and all I could think about is "we're almost done, why on earth would I want to start over?" No matter how many times I tried to talk myself out of it my heart wanted what it wanted. I desired to have a little piece of myself in this world.

One day I came home from work, sat my husband down, and expressed to him my newfound desire of wanting a baby. Total shock and confusion came across his face. He was speechless. He had this look that read, "who are you and what have you done with my wife?" After taking a moment to digest the conversation, he finally responded with excitement. We had just bought a new home, and we were both settling into our careers.

Over the next several weeks we started having more and more conversations on if we were seriously going to have a baby. We began mapping out our plan on how we intended on moving forward.

I am a very calculated person. I'm talking life mapped out on a spreadsheet type of calculated. Everything must make sense before making any sudden decisions. So, after careful considerations and numerous conversations about our goals and desires, we decided to move forward with having a baby. I decided I would discuss my plans and desires of conceiving at my upcoming appointment with my **OBGYN**. While at my appointment, my doctor informed me of the importance of using an ovulation kit while trying to conceive. Before that, I had no idea what an ovulation kit was. She informed me an ovulation kit (also known as an ovulation test) detects the presence of Luteinizing Hormone (LH) in your urine. When you get a positive test, it means that it is the perfect time to conceive. What some may not understand is the older you get the harder it is to get pregnant. The prime years to get pregnant are late teens thru mid-twenties. Your body at this age is at its most fertile stage and is considered easier to get pregnant. Which worried me considering I was almost thirty. My doctor told me to come back and visit her in six months if we were having difficulty conceiving.

I was gleaming with joy at the thought of having a baby. I was so excited that I stopped on the way home to buy ovulation kits and a pregnancy test. But after six long months of trying, with positive ovulation testing, we were advised to see a fertility specialist. My stomach dropped, FERTILITY SPECIALIST. I fell into a bit of a depression wondering what was wrong with me. Why wasn't I able to conceive? I started to think back on all those years I took motherhood for granted. I was wondering why pregnancy for us wasn't happening. Everywhere I turned, couples were announcing their pregnancies. Although I was truly happy for them, a piece of me was broken. I wanted to experience that same joy for myself. I was becoming hopeless.

PSA

Let's talk about something important concerning conception. Many people have a bad habit of asking couples when they are going to have kids. I have been guilty of this a time or two also. This question may be insensitive and painful for couples to answer. Although it's not coming from a malicious place it is improper to ask a woman when she plans on having a baby. Some women don't plan on having kids, but others just can't. As much as they try, cry, beg and plea they will never be able to bear a child. It can be a sensitive subject matter and your asking is a reminder of their invisible bleeding wound.

Simply put: Don't ask women about their plans on bearing children.

Over the next couple of months, we were sent to see a fertility specialist. We had several different tests ran to determine why I was having difficulty conceiving. My first test was a general pelvic exam. I also had an ultrasound to look at my uterus and ovaries. My husband then had to submit a sample of his best swimmers. Finally, I had blood work done to check my hormone levels and to check for genetic disorders.

After everything came back normal, I was then sent to the hospital for a "special x-ray test" called a hysterosalpingogram (HSG). This test helps to see if your fallopian tubes are open or blocked. AGAIN, everything came back normal, but I was still unable to get pregnant. We then had an appointment to discuss our options: medication to help me ovulate or the possibility of In Vitro Fertilization (IVF). That was a devastating blow for me. I found myself in a bit of a depressed funk. I felt less than a woman because I was unable to produce a child.

At this point, it had been more than a year trying to conceive. I was getting positive results on my ovulation test and still not pregnant yet. I felt at this point I should try medication to help with conception. I called my fertility specialist and was prescribed Femara. This drug would help induce my ovulation and increase my chances of getting pregnant. I was educated on how to use it for my next cycle. While waiting for my cycle to come on to start my ovulation medication, I started feeling this pain in my uterus and I first considered it to be menstrual cramps. But something deep down told me it wasn't. I went to Dr. Google to figure out what this could be. I came across the term implantation and I KNEW that was the feeling I was having. Implantation is the attaching of the fertilized egg into the uterus wall. Some can feel it and others can't.

About a week later I started to get very nauseous. Let's just say, I've never been more excited in my life to be sick. I KNEW in my heart I was pregnant! But how, I was scheduled to start my first round of ovulation medication the following month. So, I wanted a test to confirm my speculation. I needed to lay my nerves to rest. I woke up one morning went into the bathroom (before my husband got up for work) and took a test. As I watched the two lines come up my eyes started to water and before you know it...I was crying tears of pure joy! I was jumping up and down and screaming quietly because I didn't want to wake him up. I had to plan a cute and creative way to tell him the news! I couldn't believe, after everything we endured, WE WERE FINALLY PREGNANT.

"Meeting people at my fertility doctor's office who are going through the same things I'm going through, I thought, 'Why not share my story?' It's really been emotional."

-Kim Kardashian

PART 2

PREGNANCY

Now that I laid out the back story let's get into all the shit no one talks about when it comes to pregnancy and motherhood.

I found myself being ashamed to say I was going through some of the issues I was going through during pregnancy, early postpartum, and even well into motherhood. But why should I be ashamed I couldn't be the only mother going through these situations. Out of all the women I knew before me that were mothers none of them spoke about any of the things I was experiencing. Why did it have to be so taboo? So, I decided to write about all my personal experiences to let the

21

next mother know, that I also went through what you went through and it's okay to talk about it. You're not alone it doesn't have to be such an off-limits topic. So, let's get into it:

Morning sickness

Not even close to what it sounds like. Morning sickness doesn't just affect you in the morning it actually occurs at any time of the day or night for that fact. It's caused by the increase of hormones in your body in the first trimester. If you're like me, I was looking forward to the end of the first trimester to start feeling better. Halfway into my second trimester, I realized that I was probably going to be sick my entire pregnancy. For some women like myself, I experienced Hyperemesis Gravidarum (HG) which is an extreme form of morning sickness. Every part of the house I went to I had to carry my "vomit bucket" with me that my lovely husband bought me. There was a time where I couldn't make it to the bathroom in time and he had to clean it up. Let's just say that was his last time cleaning it up hence the bucket.

I was sick up until the day I gave birth causing me to be very dehydrated my entire pregnancy. There are many forms of medication to help even a pump that supplies anti-nausea medicine which has an injection site on your stomach. Now that was no fun, I am not a fan of needles, and having to self-inject was miserable and my stomach was so tender from all the injection spots. My hyperemesis was so bad the medication did not help but just because it didn't work for me doesn't mean it may not work for you. O goodness I was so sick I made a vow to never get pregnant again and told my husband he needed to get a vasectomy.

Food Aversions

Once the morning sickness started the cravings and food aversions followed shortly afterward. Food aversion is when certain foods that you once loved you can no longer stomach the taste or smell of them. I ate relatively healthy before I got pregnant and now, I could not even handle the sight of fruits and vegetables anymore. I could eat something one day and the next I could not. My cravings were so random and hard to keep up with. I once requested chitterlings; I don't even eat that on special holidays, so that was shocking for everyone around me. For the first trimester, I got cravings so bad in the middle of the night, I would be up for hours constantly eating trying to curb my hunger pains. I finally made it easier on myself and I started sleeping on the living room couch, to be closer to the kitchen.

Sleepiness

I was not aware of how much work the body takes to create a baby. What we can't see early on is that our body is working overtime. It's constantly changing physically, which causes us to be extremely tired throughout our pregnancy but especially during the first trimester. Our hormones are going full throttle and the major one that causes you sleepiness is Progesterone. Our hormones are also affecting our blood sugar and blood pressure which can cause overall tiredness. During this time, I listened to my body and when she said sleep, I SLEPT. Although you may not feel like you're doing a lot don't feel guilty. I read once where "Pregnancy pushes the body nearly as much as extreme sports"

Round Ligament Pain

So, as I entered my second trimester my belly was heavy and uncomfortable. I would have these feelings of aches and pain on both sides and even under my abdomen. Sometimes I would experience what felt like a sharp, jabbing pain, and other times it would just be a dull cramp. I remember being at work and a co-worker asking what was wrong. I guess the grimacing look on my face and constant holding of my lower belly gave it away. As I described my pain, she explained I was experiencing round ligament pain or what some may describe as "growing pains." As your uterus grows your ligaments that are attached to your uterus for support stretches to carry the weight. My co-worker informed me that wearing a belly band would help in aiding in the support of my increasingly heavy belly. I also found sitting down, kicking my feet up and hydrating helped a lot too.

Low Iron

I went to lay down one day because I was feeling very fatigued and exhausted. As I laid there, I realized I was feeling very weak and faint. Lifting my arm seemed like a task of its own. I knew something wasn't right. I called my doctor to inform her of my symptoms, she recommended I come in to get some blood work done to find out what was going on. I got a phone call the next day saying that my iron was low, and I was very anemic. Low iron means red blood cells are unable to carry oxygen throughout the body. I was informed I needed to start taking iron supplements daily. I started on one pill a day and eventually upgraded to three pills a day. The prescription supplements weren't helping much so I was advised to start Vitron-C. What I learned is that iron is best absorbed with vitamin c: ie the Vitron-C or with a glass of orange juice. I also started incorporating iron-rich foods into my diet to help increase my levels. Some examples are:

- Liver

- Beets

- Green leafy vegetables

- Beans

Gestational Diabetes

So, thankfully I never had gestational diabetes, but I did have a scare. That's the last thing I needed on top of dealing with anemia. I failed my first glucose test and was told I had to do a three-hour fasting test. That's where you can't eat anything after midnight and the next morning your blood is drawn every hour for three hours after drinking a highly concentrated sugary drink. Luckily for me, I passed the second go-round. Had I not I would have had to check my blood sugar before my meals by a finger prick. If levels weren't controlled by diet, then I could have been on medication such as Metformin or Insulin. Unlike regular diabetes, gestational diabetes is caused by your body not being able to produce insulin due to your placenta's hormones. Gestational diabetes occurs during pregnancy and usually resolves on its own afterward.

Constipation/Gas

So, if you know then you know. Iron supplements and constipation goes hand in hand. I had no idea what I was in store for. I didn't realize it would make me constipated! I learned that taking MiraLAX and adding more fiber to my diet helped. Now to add insult to injury my husband and I are very cute about our gas. I was so embarrassed to let one go around him but gas while pregnant is no joke. When you have to let go you just have to let go and often. So, this particular time I had gas while we were in the car together and I tried to just "hold it." Nope, the universe would not let me be great. I shamefully said "I have gas & I can't hold it I'm sorry," he said he understood laughed, and let the window down.

Hemorrhoids

Hemorrhoids are uncomfortable to talk about and most importantly to deal with but are quite common during pregnancy and postpartum. If you were lucky enough to not have experienced them like I did and don't know what hemorrhoids are, they are varicose veins in the rectum. It's caused by the pressure of your uterus, increased blood flow, constipation, and pushing during delivery.

Staying hydrated and drinking plenty of water is vital during pregnancy for many reasons. One is to help aid in regular bowel movements. It's important to stay regular and increase your fiber intake to avoid constipation. I'm here to let you know that postpartum hemorrhoids are no fun either. Witch hazel, ice packs, and lidocaine spray are going to be your friend. It helps with the uncomfortableness and soothes the pain.

Always Hot

I was not prepared to be so hot. I figured since most of my months pregnant were during winter months I missed all of the dreaded summer pregnancy talks I've heard. But I was still so hot that I would walk around in a sports bra and shorts on most days. I would go to sleep with the AC in the 60's and two fans blowing on me while my poor husband was freezing and sleeping with his head under the cover. This happens because of the surge in hormones and the heart is pumping an increased amount of blood and your blood vessels dilate bringing them closer to the skin causing you to feel hot. Contrary to what I went through some may feel cold all the time.

Constantly on the Go

I always had the urge to pee as much as I would try to hold it my bladder was not taking no for an answer. It felt like my baby was just sitting directly on my bladder and the slightest kick would send me wobbling to the bathroom. I already have horrible insomnia, but I learned pregnant women don't get much sleep because we're always in the bathroom. I used to sleep on the side of the bed that was farthest from the bathroom, but my husband and I decided to make a switch for my convenience. (Actually, I told him what was going to happen, and he gave me a side-eye, annoyed gestured and switched) As many of you know it's pretty much an unspoken rule about how couples have their own side of the bed!

Sleeping on your left side

Like I mentioned before pregnant women are always tired and a man may think we just sleep a lot, but a night's sleep is not as "restful" as they may think. Aside from the constant urge to urinate, I had the hardest time sleeping at night because I would normally sleep on my stomach or back. So, when I learned I had to sleep on my side I was like wtf!! Like who comfortably sleeps on their side and why can I not at least sleep on my back. It's important the further along you get to sleep on your right-side. As your uterus grows and gets heavier it weighs on your vital organs and a major blood vessel, inferior vena cava (IVC), that maintains proper blood flow to mom and baby. Ironically outside of pregnancy I am now a side sleeper, my left side to be exact. Sleeping on my side also caused hip pain, mostly my right hip. So, sleeping with a body pillow and pillow between your knees could help a lot with proper alignment to make sleeping a bit more comfortable.

Loose joints

I remember strolling down the hallway at work and someone making a comment about my walk. I didn't even realize I had started wobbling. I just remember feeling heavy and winded even during a short walk. That night I came home to a special meal cooked by my mother-in-law. Who by the way would drive in town just to cook me a meal since I had a hard time keeping food down. After dinner, I went to sleep and woke up to a quiet house to empty my bladder of course. While returning to bed, I went to lift my hip and leg to get in bed, but my knee popped out of place which sent chills down my spine. I was in so much pain and let out a loud moan because I didn't want to startle everyone and create panic. My husband woke up not knowing what to do and I couldn't explain because I was in so much pain, so I just moaned. My husband helped get my leg straightened out to relieve the pain. After I got settled in bed, we laughed so hard and all I could think of is my mother-in-law who was in the next room may have thought we were having sex. The next morning my mother-in-law never made mention and neither did I. What I learned during pregnancy that there is an abundance of different hormones working together to prepare you for delivery. One of them in particular is called Relaxin. Relaxin loosens your muscles, joints, and ligaments so your pelvis is ready for delivery hence the wobble in my walk and dislocated knee.

Baby Brain

Baby brain sometimes referred to as "Placenta Brain" is what we say when we become forgetful or absentminded during pregnancy. I remember one day being too sick to cook so I ordered takeout. When asked for my address I couldn't remember it. I drew a complete blank. I had to ask my stepdaughter who stood in amazement that as grown as I was, I couldn't remember my own address. If it wasn't for her help, I would have probably sent our dinner to one of our neighbors. I also noticed I had become dyslexic; I never had this problem before. I would send emails and text messages with so many spelling errors it blew my mind that I couldn't spell simple words. That particular year our families came together for Thanksgiving at our house and I drew a turkey with the words "Gobble til you Wobble" on the chalkboard or I thought I did. After everyone had eaten my sister-in-law realized my error and pointed it out to everyone that I actually wrote "Gooble til you Wooble" and let's just say I have to re-live this spelling error every Thanksgiving now.

Increased Sex drive

Now, this may be too much information for some but if I'm laying it all out there, then let's talk about everything. My sex drive increased during pregnancy and my husband was not complaining. I remember my libido being super intense and couldn't understand where all this extra energy was coming from. What I learned is that the spike in our hormones and increased blood flow to the genital areas and breasts leads to heightened sexual desires. Some women have the opposite effect with a decreased sex drive or none at all. Some causes of that may be due to sickness and fatigue. Hormones affect us all differently. I was very apprehensive at first about having sex during pregnancy. Working in the labor and delivery unit I have seen women come in time and time again from contracting after having sex. I just did not want to be that patient, how embarrassing could that be to say, "Sex sent me to the ER." It's ok it happens. Sperm combined with mom's hormones released from an orgasm can in some cases soften the cervix and cause contractions. Sex generally is safe during pregnancy but in some instances can cause premature labor. If you are concerned talk with your doctor first.

What to Take to the Hospital

The time had finally arrived for me to be induced and meet my little miracle baby! My doctor provided us a list of essential items to bring to the hospital that I thought I would share. Thank goodness she did because with my baby brain I would have been sending my husband to go back and forth to get things. I added a few things of my own to the list:

-Gown & Robe

-Hair product

-House slippers/Shower shoes

-Mom and baby going home outfit

-Personal Hygiene products

-Vaseline (if you're having a boy)

-Games and electronics ie: card games in case you get bored

"If I had my life to live over, instead of wishing away nine months of pregnancy, I'd have cherished every moment and realized that the wonderment growing inside me was the only chance in life to assist God in a miracle." —

Erma Bombeck

PART 3

LABOR AND

DELIVERY

The day had finally arrived to meet my bundle of joy and I was overwhelmed with emotions. My induction date was pushed back a couple of days due to the Labor and Delivery unit not having any available beds. We got a call at six o'clock in the morning, asking if we could be there by nine that morning to start my induction. I was excited and nervous at the same time. We decided to wait until the delivery to learn the sex of our baby. So, all I could think about was if I was having a boy or a girl and snuggling with my new love. But then I started to feel severe anxiety. I started thinking about the pain of labor. I made it to the Women's Center and got situated into my room. Shortly after getting changed my nurse came in and put the blood pressure cuff on and got me hooked up to the fetal monitor. She asked me some questions, proceeded to draw lab work, put in an IV, and hooked me up to fluids. The nurse left and I turned to my husband and stepdaughter who both had excitement written all over their face and I gave them a warm smile.

Two hours had passed, and the nurse returned with a medicine cup saying it was time for the Pitocin. Pitocin is a man-made form of the natural hormone Oxytocin.

Pitocin is given to stimulate your uterus to contract. It is often said that contractions due to Pitocin are more intense compared to natural contractions. I have nothing to compare it to, I can say without a doubt, my contractions were pure hell! I told myself pre-labor that I was going to go as long as I could without an epidural. Not because I necessarily wanted to, but because my mom and mother-in-law did it. Surely if they could go without one I could too, right?! On the other hand, I could also hear my sisters-in-law saying, "you better get the epidural!" About two hours into my contractions, I asked my nurse for something to help with the pain. She returned with morphine. Although it did help, it did not last long. Another hour had passed, and my contractions were so painful that I just knew I dilated a few centimeters. My nurse came in to check me and proceeded to inform me that I only dilated half a centimeter. I wanted to cry! THREE hours of labor and basically, I was unchanged. I remember the nurse asking if I wanted an epidural. I don't remember the curse words I used, but the nurse was back shortly setting me up for the procedure. I completely disregarded what the women in my life did before me. They created epidurals for a reason, and I was going to use it!

The CRNA came in and I was so relieved to see him. As I sat up to get my epidural, he told me that it would help, but it would not take all the pain away. That was the last thing I wanted to hear. What do you mean it won't take all the pain away? My anxiety spiked because I just couldn't imagine being able to deal with another contraction.

The epidural stung, but it wasn't unbearable. I felt it was worth it. I no longer felt my contractions. THANK GOD! With the epidural in place, I was less tense and started to relax. In return, my body was able to dilate. For the next six hours, labor started moving fast. By eight p.m. my nurse came and put the oxygen mask on me. She started to roll me from side to side. She informed me that my babies' heart rate had dropped, and she needed to bring it back up. Tears rolled down my face because working in the field I've seen times like this turn into emergency c-sections. I was shaking uncontrollably at this point and looked over and saw fear in the eyes of my family. In midst of her getting my baby's heart rate back up, I could hear her on the phone telling my doctor "It's Time, she's complete."

Things were moving so fast I felt like I was in the twilight zone! The room was filling up with staff members prepping the room for delivery. It was such an "out of body" experience. It was completely different now that I was the patient. I was nervous, but at the same time felt secure with my nurse. She was really on her shit. I knew my doctor was at a special ceremony dinner with her daughter and felt bad she would have to leave. But somehow, she was in the delivery room within thirty mins flat gowned and gloved telling me to push.

The time had arrived for me to start pushing and I couldn't wait to meet my baby! All I remember is hearing the count down and being told to push. I still couldn't feel anything since I got that great epidural. I was doing my best to "push", but I couldn't tell if I was doing it correctly or not. But apparently, I was doing it right, because with a total of two pushes I was told "stop the baby is out". My doctor handed her to me, and I burst out into tears. The doctor asked if I saw the gender, but I was crying so much I couldn't even see clearly.

That evening I delivered a baby girl weighing in at 6 lbs 7oz. named Ava Love. I held her all night and just watched her sleep. As sleepy as I was, it was so peaceful to watch over her. Life felt so unreal. I couldn't process that I had just brought a child into this world. I was now the mother of a beautiful little girl. To be honest, I had to get used to saying my "daughter", it sounded so foreign to me.

It was now time for her first feeding, but I had trouble breastfeeding due to her having a lip and tongue tie. A lip and tongue tie is when the membrane under the tongue (the frenulum) is too tight. It makes it difficult for the baby to latch on to the breast and causes them difficulty swallowing. Thankfully, we had an attentive nurse who noticed that I was in so much pain and caught the problem early. We had an appointment set up with a highly recommended Pediatric Dentist the day we left the hospital. We drove an hour away to have an easy laser procedure done to remove the ties.

"Before you were conceived, I wanted you. Before you were born, I loved you. Before you were here an hour, I would die for you. This is the miracle of Mother's Love." —

Maureen Hawkins

PART 4

MOTHERHOOD

We were finally home from the hospital and I couldn't have been happier being in my own bed. For some reason the reality had not quite set in that I had a baby. Life was truly about to change. I wish I would have known what to expect so I could have understood the changes I was going through. I started to feel completely inadequate. During the first couple of months, I had times when I felt like a complete failure as a parent. If I would have known that other mothers also felt gloomy during this stage, I would not have felt so alone. The reason I wanted to talk about the things I went through in such an open manner is not

scare new moms, but to inform them. All the feelings you may feel, you should know, you are not alone.

Visitors

I decided that we wouldn't have any visitors for Ava's first six weeks. We didn't want her to get sick during the flu season and considered waiting until her immune system was more developed. Now I know that is unorthodox, but I'm not the type to do things by status quo. Risk aversion was the main catalyst in making this decision. It's ok to set your boundaries and not feel guilty about it. I never intended to hurt anyone's feelings, but I knew what I wanted for my baby. Even after my six-week rule, I wasn't big on having a lot of visitors. The baby receives all of the love, attention and affection of family and friends. Rarely do people take the time to check on the parents. It may be the parents that need a little extra love and attention. So many changes are occurring mentally and physically for them especially mom.

POSTPARTUM DEPRESSION & ANXIETY

After having my daughter, I struggled with postpartum depression (PPD) as many women do. Postpartum depression is a type of depression that usually occurs after childbirth. It emerges due to the combination of hormonal changes, stress, fatigue, and the physical and physiological changes that comes with motherhood. Statically 50-75% of women experience mood swings or sadness. This is also known as "baby blues." Traditionally it only lasts 2 weeks or so. Studies show that 15% of these women go on to develop postpartum depression. I often wondered to myself WHY IS THIS TOPIC NOT

TALKED ABOUT MORE!

I've never heard it talked about amongst family and friends. My first time learning about it was while I was going through it. I learned people never want to expose their weaknesses. They want to appear as if they have it all together. But this topic should be talked about more. Just because you're dealing with motherhood differently than other mothers, doesn't make you less adequate. Postpartum depression hit me about a month after having my daughter. I was so upset that I had the overwhelming feeling of being sad all the time. I was unable to experience joy. One day, my husband asked if I was ok. The expression on my face must have told him I was not. I began crying out of frustration. I was exhausted! I was juggling two kids and felt like I couldn't even do the basic things for myself. It was a struggle for me to find the time to make food let alone find the time to eat it. At the time, only my husband knew of the difficulty I was having transitioning into motherhood. Ironically, I didn't feel comfortable talking to anyone about it. For the first couple of months after delivery, I didn't want to be around anyone. I was going through so many changes at once. I remember my best friend was getting married and I was so worried that I would not be ready to be in a social environment so soon. I was so depressed. To add insult to injury, I was self-conscious about the way my body looked. I was stressed thinking I would not be able to fit into my bridal dress. This was going to be one of the happiest days of her life, yet I was so mentally distressed. I was able to push through my emotions and make it to her wedding. I was not doing as good of a job as I thought I was of masking my feelings. My best friend kept asking if I was ok. I felt heartbroken that I was unable to be a better version of myself at that moment.

Tragically five months after my daughter was born, I fell into a deeper depression. My brother passed away, and I was at the lowest point I had ever been in my life. Realizing I couldn't shake the funk, I decided it was time to talk to my doctor and implement some lifestyle changes. It wasn't until my daughter was going on 1 ½, that I felt a shift. I began feeling better. By my daughter's second birthday I noticed I was feeling like myself again. During this time, I began opening up more with loved ones and even posting the

71

topic on social media. I began talking about my difficulties juggling motherhood and Postpartum depression. I got a few responses of "me too!" I got a ton of private messages expressing that they also had similar situations. I was amazed at how ALONE so many people felt. Why is postpartum depression so taboo to discuss? I plan on breaking that cycle by speaking up. I want to let women know that it is ok to be vulnerable. I want to use my voice to inform women and men of the signs to look for because as we know motherhood/parenthood doesn't come with a manual.

SEPARATION ANXIETY

On top of postpartum depression, I had maternal separation anxiety. I know, I know, normally you only think of infants and young children when it comes to separation anxiety. Many mothers can develop it also. My separation anxiety issues were like adding gasoline on a fire that was already out of control. I was crying because I needed a break and was exhausted and fatigued. But I felt an overwhelming sense of anxiousness and guilt when I didn't have her. Leaving my husband to watch her made me feel so uncomfortable. My husband would offer me breaks but I would find myself going to the living room with them just so that I could be in the same room as her while I slept. My husband is a wonderful partner and father. But for some reason, I just felt like no one could take care of her the way I could. It was hard for me to leave the house for "me time" because I didn't want to be without her.

SLEEP DEPRIVATION

As all mothers know, it is not easy taking care of a newborn. We often neglect our own needs. Sleep deprivation is common. Waking up every three hours for feedings, diaper changes, or comforting a newborn is exhausting. It doesn't help that for a lot of babies the mother is the only source of milk. A normal sleep cycle would consist of seven to nine hours a night. Researchers found that new moms were averaging between three to four hours a night. What helped a lot was sleeping when she slept. I would turn my phone on silent and catch a nap with her. As much I considered myself superwoman I wasn't. Being sleep deprived makes you more at risk of postpartum depression. I began delegating tasks and responsibilities so that I did not feel more overwhelmed than I was.

UNABLE TO SETTLE CRYING BABY

Dealing with an upset baby can be stressful because you have no clue exactly what they are trying to communicate. It's a big game of "guess what's wrong." I found that the 5 S's that I was taught from a lactation nurse worked for her: 1. Swaddling 2. Side/stomach position 3. Shushing 4. Swinging and 5. Sucking. For a long time, I had no idea that she was colicky. What I thought I was doing to help calm her was not working because she was crying from an upset stomach. One night I had to rush out to the store to get gas medicine to help calm her down. I learned that she did not like a wet diaper and as soon as she would pee, she would cry to get it off her. It took some time, but I eventually started to learn what her different cries meant.

BREASTFEEDING

As I mentioned before I had trouble breastfeeding due to her having a lip tie and tongue tie. We were unable to get that initial connection in the hospital. I felt I didn't know what I was doing. I was so determined to breastfeed because I felt it was best for her. I would set up meetings with lactation nurses to get assistance. We were still having a difficult time latching. So, I was strictly pumping my milk for her which was draining. I was overproducing milk, and the pump could only do so much. Unlike breastfeeding, the pump doesn't have the same suction to draw milk out of the glands and ducts. Which caused me to develop clogged ducts not once but twice. This led me to have mastitis. Mastitis is breast swelling and pain that causes fever and chills and is usually treated with a round of antibiotics. It was a really difficult decision when I decided to give up breastfeeding. I felt like I was failing her by going to formula. But we just weren't successful with latching and I couldn't bear the pain of getting mastitis again. What I learned is a full baby is a happy baby and it didn't matter if it was formula or breastmilk.

POSTPARTUM HEALING

Talking about what I was going through was a start to healing my depression. I was determined to start feeling better. I spoke with my doctor and she recommended that I get started on an anti-depressant to help balance my emotions out. I was leery at first, but she explained to me that it wouldn't be long term. The analogy she gave me was, "when you break your arm you have to put it in a cast to heal right? Well this is the same you need help healing." That gave me comfort and has stuck with me ever since. I also got back into things I enjoyed doing such as yoga and meditation. Studies have found that yoga and meditation can reduce the impact of stress and be self-soothing. Getting out of the house alone more helped as well. I began taking more time for myself to do things that didn't involve the kids. Such as getting my nails done again, going to eat, and getting massages. I also started implementing Self Care Sundays where I would spend time alone to read, do an adult coloring book, spa bath with candles and music, or simply have a glass of wine. I realized the importance of making time for **MYSELF!**

"The moment a child is born, the mother is also born. She never existed before. The woman existed, but the mother, never. A mother is something absolutely new." —

Rajneesh

During the worst of my postpartum depression I couldn't imagine going through another pregnancy but recently I find myself sitting in solitude rubbing my growing belly. I pass time daydreaming about my son's arrival soon. Through it all I loved being a mother to my daughter so much I was willing to do it all over. Again, I have an overwhelming feeling of pure joy. For once, I felt like I figured it out. I figured out my purpose in life! I found what motivates and drives me to get up every day and love what I do. As my husband walked into the room I asked him what was his "Purpose in life?" he stared off in thought like he normally does when we have our deep thought-provoking conversations and said, "That's a good question I never really thought about it." He then asked in return "do you know what your purpose in life is?" I replied without hesitation "Being a Mother!" I had a powerful revelation. "Wow, I was born for this. I was born to be someone's Mom!" It's just so ironic to me because for so many years I thought I never wanted kids.

Out of the many things, everyone failed to mention to me about motherhood the biggest was that I never truly understood what love was beforehand. Don't get me wrong, when I say I love you to love ones I one hundred percent mean it. But what I have learned is the love I have for my child is something different, so complex, it's truly difficult to explain. I was in love at the very moment I saw those two lines come up on the pregnancy test. It was a feeling I had never felt before. That love grew and developed over the course of nine months. Faint butterflies then turned into rib kicks. I would then fall more in love when I would listen to her heartbeat during the ultrasound appointments. I would daydream about what she would look like. What her voice would sound like. How I would raise her and protect her! Then when I set eyes on her I was overwhelmed with happiness. As I held her admiring her beauty, I realized I never experienced a love like this. Two years after having her and being so enchanted by her presence, I decided I wanted to experience this all over again. Humbly, I had to eat my words when I said I wouldn't have anymore!

Although I get exhausted, and I have moments where I cry, there isn't anything in this world that makes me happier than being a mother.

Made in the USA
Middletown, DE
10 July 2022